QUICK MEAL REPEAT

A THOROUGH GUIDE ON POSTPONING INTERMITTENT FASTING, RATHER THAN DENYING IT

LILLIAN J. OGLE

The counsel of the reader's doctor or other medical professionals is not intended to be replaced by the information in this book. Before beginning, halting and or altering the dosage of any drug you are taking, you should visit a medical practitioner about any health-related issues, especially if you have pre-existing problems. Each reader is completely in charge of their own healthcare decisions. Any negative impacts that readers may allege to have encountered, whether directly or indirectly, as a result of the information in this book, are not the responsibility of the author or the publisher.

TABLE OF CONTENT

PRODUCTION

It is a well-known fact that America has a weight issue. As per the CDC, almost three-diggings of us are fat or fat. However, more than 160 million Americans are on a tight eating routine at some random time, and we drop further than $70 billion each time on attractive weight reduction plans, supplements and other pound-slipping measures. That recommends that horrible weight is difficult — yet it's not outside the realm of possibilities when done well. There are two keys to progress in weight reduction. The first is to find a methodology that works for you explicitly, one that causes you to feel better and keeps you inspired. The option is to take as much time as is needed practical weight reduction happens slowly however consistently.

Before you set out on your difficulty, ensure you know precisely the very thing you're attempting to accomplish. How much weight do I need to shed to be healthy? Additionally, set validated assumptions, and feasible enhancements and acquaint life changes with gradually getting fitter and keep it off. Be set to adapt your life as important to expand your odds of coming out on top.

What's the snazzy eating routine for weight reduction?

It's an inquiry into the personalities of most extreme individuals whenever they've concluded they need to shed a few pounds — what is the snazzy eating routine for weight reduction? While that is not an irrational inquiry, it regularly suggests a methodology that is lower than ideal, which is to anticipate embracing a profoundly prohibitive method of eating for some time, until the weight is lost, and returning to eating as typical. As opposed to embracing " style abstains from food, " individuals who have shed pounds — and kept it off — by and large have made a perpetual shift toward better dietary patterns. Supplanting unfortunate food varieties with sound bones — not for a long time, but rather ever — will assist you with accomplishing weight reduction while likewise offering endless different advantages. Therefore, a better set of questions may be, "What constitutes a healthy diet?"

A sound eating routine blesses normal, undressed food sources over-bundled reflections and bites. It's decent, implying that it furnishes your body with every one of the supplements and minerals it necessities to stunningly serve. It stresses industrial facility-grounded food varieties — particularly products of the soil over monster food sources. It contains a wealth of protein. It's low in sugar and sugar. It consolidates " solid fats " including fish, olive oil painting and other plant-derived materials.

There are numerous instances of solid reflections for weight reduction. For breakfast, an open-air theatre of grain pieces with cut strawberries and pecans with nonfat milk. Lunch will consist of a wheat-based lemon sandwich with veggies, an olive oil painting, and a ginger dressing. A salmon steak atop a bed of spinach for amusement.

You don't need to remove snacks to eat a solid eating routine, besides. Solid snacks for weight reduction incorporate almonds or pistachios, string refills with an apple, Greek yoghurt or a banana with nut hero worship.

Before you start your weight reduction trip, do some conceptualizing about the sorts of quality food sources you appreciate with the goal that you can have bunches of decisions as you plan your snacks. The flashback is that the in-vogue diet is the bone you'll adhere to, so don't rush out and purchase a lot of "well-being food sources " that you realize you'll have no chance to eat.

Which diet is recommended?
Nutritionists haven't identified a single diet plan as "the best." However, there are several eating habits that experts have either recommended for optimal health or have observed to be healthy when regularly practised by people all over the world. Comparative eating patterns will typically have many similarities to Western eating patterns, including a preference for whole, plant-based foods over highly processed, frequently reused foods. They will also frequently emphasize healthy fats, no added sugars, low sodium, and no refined carbohydrates.

For representation, the Mediterranean-style diet gets its name from the food varieties accessible to bright social orders situated around the Mediterranean Ocean. It vigorously underlines negligibly reused organic products, vegetables, vegetables, nuts and entire grains. It contains moderate amounts of yoghurt, garbage, tissue and fish. Olive oil painting is its essential cooking fat. Red meat and foods with added sugars are only consumed in moderation. Other than being a viable weight reduction framework, eating a Mediterranean-style diet is connected to a lower danger of heart grumblings, diabetes, wretchedness and a few types of disease.

Specialists fostered the Scramble diet(Dietary Ways to Deal with Stop Hypertension) explicitly as a heart-sound power. The blend of food types contained in the eating regimen feels to cooperate particularly to bring down circulatory strain and drop the danger of cardiovascular breakdown. The vital elements of energy are low cholesterol and impregnated fats, loads of magnesium, calcium, fibre and potassium, and almost no red meat and sugar. Usually, that is likened to a rundown of food sources closely resembling those of the Mediterranean eating routine — entire grains, vegetables, organic products, fish, tissue, nuts and olive oil painting.

As its name suggests, the Psyche diet(Mediterranean-Run diet Intercession for Neurodegenerative Deferral) was planned by Croakers to take basics from the Mediterranean and Run eat fewer carbs that sounded to give advantages to cerebrum well-being and fight off the frenzy and mental deterioration. By and by, it's genuinely equivalent to both the Mediterranean and Run, which eats less carbs, however, it puts a more grounded accentuation on rich green vegetables and berries, and a lower accentuation on leafy foods.

As of late, the Nordic eating routine has surfaced as both a weight reduction and well-being-protection diet. Grounded on Scandinavian eating designs, the Nordic eating regimen is weighty on fish, apples, pears, entire grains like rye and oats, and cold-environment vegetables including cabbage, carrots and cauliflower. Studies have upheld its utilization both in blocking stroke and in weight reduction.

What exactly do these weight-control strategies have in common? They're great overall for your heart, they all compare to normal striped food varieties and they all contain processed plant-grounded,factory-grounded dishes. Eating for your well-being — particularly your heart's well-being — by upholding fundamentals from these eating regimens is a savvy method for shedding pounds.

CHAPTER ONE

WHY FASTING IS SIGNIFICANT

Americans are continually looking for the best, most proficient way to deal with getting thinner. The eating regimen industry is extravagant subsequently. Notwithstanding, diet prevailing fashions and frenzies travel every which way, and a large number of them aren't long haul helpful. The latest eating method, discontinuous fasting, involves standard, brief diets, or times when you consume not many or no calories.

As irregular fasting acquires notoriety among superstars, it is drawing media consideration. As per advocates, it energizes weight reduction or weight support while likewise saving bulk and directing insulin levels.

Although the "IF" or "quick" diet, at times, alluded to as irregular fasting, is well known, you might have misgivings about its viability and security.

What impacts does an intermittent quick have on my body?

You consume fewer calories than expected — or none by any means — when you are quick, which brings down your everyday calorie utilization. Albeit cutting calories can help with weight reduction, it additionally influences how your body stores and consumes fat in other ways.

The pancreas secretes the chemical insulin, which changes the blood's glucose (sugar) into cell fuel. Insulin advances the aggregation of fat. At the point when you eat, your body's insulin levels rise; when you quick, they fall. Fasting can bring about lower insulin levels, which can help your body put away fat and stop further fat stockpiling.

What varieties of discontinuous fasting are there?

Consuming your calories rapidly is a part of discontinuous fasting. There are various irregular eating designs, so it's basic to pick the one that is best for your body, level of activity, and lifestyle. The following are two popular decisions:

The 16:8 Eating routine

The 16:8 eating routine includes fasting for 16 hours every day and consuming each of your calories during an 8-hour window. Various individuals who follow this 16-hour presto eat 2 reflections between early afternoon and 8 pm, however, you can adjust the 8-hour window to suit your life, practice propensities and plan for getting work done. With this choice, plan your eating so the development of the quick happens during your ordinary resting hours. This will assist you with abstaining from feeling void during your waking hours.

The 5:2 Eating regimen

Another famous choice is the 5:2 eating regimen, which includes 5 days of typical eating and 2 days of eating around 500-600 calories each day. The 5:2 eating regimen gives you the firmness to pick the 2 fasting days that turn out in vogue for you, for however long they're isolated by somewhere around one typical eating day.

What would be a good idea for me to eat and drink for a quick while?

During a quick, you can hydrate and other sans-calorie beverages, like tea or dark espresso. various individuals likewise drink bone stock, which contains supplements that help your body during a quick. Drinking fluids additionally assist with balancing weakness and look at hunger.

In any case, you ought to focus on low-calorie, high-protein and high-fibre food varieties that will assist you with remaining full, Assuming you're following a discontinuous fasting design that includes binding your calories on quick days.

What would it be a good idea for me to eat when I'm not slimming down?

Without a doubt when you're not eating less junk food, it's as yet vital to cover how various calories you devour and pick quality food varieties. avaricious during your non-fasting ages could interrupt the advantages of fasting and may for sure prompt weight gain.

Is irregular fasting safe?

Irregular fasting is one of the various instruments that can assist you with accomplishing your well-being assumptions, whether they incorporate getting more fit or controlling insulin circumstances. When done properly and securely, irregular fasting can assist with diminishing your general calorie input and may prompt weight reduction. In any case, discontinuous fasting isn't the best thing in the world for everybody.

Before you begin, check with your medical care supplier to ensure discontinuous fasting is a protected choice for you. You shouldn't attempt discontinuous fasting on the off chance that you:

- Have low glucose
- Are pregnant or nursing
- Have a past filled with eating infections
- Are light or at a typical weight

In any case, it's smart to counsel an enrolled dietitian about a discontinuous fasting plan, If your croaker says irregular fasting is ok for you. An enlisted dietitian can assist you with creating solid, reasonable eating examples and give direction about the food varieties that will give you the energy your body needs.

During irregular fasting, it's essential to focus on how you feel. You might feel unfilled and somewhat more vulnerable than typical from the start, however, you ought to adjust your eating example and converse with your medical services supplier assuming that you witness outrageous appetite, feel faint, or foster different side effects like migraines each time you gormandize.

Discontinuous fasting can be modified to accommodate your novel necessities. In any case, joining it with a solid eating routine and exercise will assist you with accomplishing your wellness assumptions sooner. What's more, similarly as with any life-altering event, moving toward irregular fasting with a sound station and looking for direction from a decent medical services provider is significant.

CHAPTER TWO

KEEPING IMPACTS CLEAN SPEEDY

Outrageous weight reduction isn't an item we suggest, however, there are kicks off to start weight reasonably and steadily.

Speedy weight reduction can sound captivating. That is particularly obvious when styling diets and virtual entertainment cause it to feel more practical than it is to drop 10 pounds in 10 days. As a matter of fact," yo gorging" or" weight cycling" is related to an expanded danger of death. The variety is, for various individuals, it's difficult to shed pounds for a heap of reasons, including life stage, body piece, actual effort, hereditary qualities and chemicals, among different elements. Besides, weight isn't the end all and is only one of a few factors that influence our general well-being.

Outrageous calorie limitation and unnecessary practising are wares our nourishment and wellness specialists would in no way suggest for well-being reasons, yet they additionally note that you will most likely restore all of your weight energetically than you lost it assuming you attempt those methodologies. Getting thinner by consummating your general eating regimen and life is without doubt the best approach.

In any case, numerous solid tips hold for virtually us all in all cases — and they're over-simplifications that we can try starting at present Assuming you are searching for manageable weight reduction.

Tips for Safe Weight Reduction

1. Up your veggie input.
Instead of keeping various food sources and nutrition types, focus on integrating a cornucopia of wholesome food sources that you can add to your eating regimen to advance general well-being and weight activity. The water and fibre in yield add volume to dishes and are normally low in fat and calories however supplement thick and stuffing. You can deliver lower-calorie exhibitions of delicious dishes by changing out cutting-edge calorie constituents for foods grown from the ground. assume cauliflower rice instead of firm white rice or do 50/50. In any case, you're in good shape for more well-being, Assuming you guess about making any

considerable veggies(something like 50 of anything that you're having).

2. make a superior breakfast.

A reasonable breakfast, one that is heaped with fibre, protein, and sound fats, meeting up in a delicious dish — will reexamine your day, particularly assuming you're by and by skipping it and nevertheless wind up flopping to focus on a solid life. Skipping breakfast might affect your yearning chemicals hitherto in the day, prompting you to feel" ridiculously hungry" in the fall which makes it harder to shun enormous parts or jones for tacky and refined carb food varieties. The snazzy, heartiest morning meals are ones that will top you off, keep you fulfilled, and fight off Jones hitherto in the day. Mean to eat anyplace somewhere in the range of 350 and 500 calories for your morning wreck, and ensure you are including a wellspring of extra protein in addition to filling fat(assume eggs, slight Greek yoghurt, nuts, or nut wool) fibre (veggies, natural product, or 100 entire grains). Beginning your day with a glucose-settling blend of supplements will assist you with thinning down.

3. Drinks with a skirt.

We simply don't feel overflowing with liquid calories in the same way that we do with real food. A stadium of veggie- and protein-pressed mix parties is far more satisfying than drinking a juice or caramel espresso drink. Avoiding crappy drinks is frequently the easiest way to get in shape physically. As a bonus, it's wonderful for effects like heart health and diabetes prevention as well. Include your juice, soft drink, sweetened espresso, tea, and cocktail contributions. However, if you consume all of those alcoholic beverages during the day, you will have consumed roughly 800 more calories by accident and will still feel hungry. (Important fact: alcohol may inhibit the breakdown of fat, making it more difficult for you to absorb those calories.)

4. Get going.

Development of any sort can be a genuinely valuable weight activity instrument. Strolling is an extraordinary, reasonable choice that bears no repetitive spa outfit except for a decent support of kicks. A new report showed that individuals who strolled 8,200 different ways each day were less inclined to become fat and experience the ill effects of significant burdensome objections and other constant well-being-related conditions. consequently, think about strolling for weight reduction and better by and large well-being.

Likewise, strength stations fabricated an extra muscle towel, which consumes further calories — at work or rest — 24 hours every day, seven days per week. The further extra muscle you have, the more energetically you will thin down.

How would you start your strength training? Try a few boards, kneeling push-ups, a lot of syllables, or hits. Use your free weights to firmly perform basic bicep curls or rear arm muscle expansions at home or the office. If you like, incorporate some new stomach, arm, back, and leg movements. Only three to four times a week of strength training can result in a rapid improvement in weight loss as well as a variety of mix, dependability, and stance.

5. Eat carefully.

Decelerating down to focus on impacts like the taste, surfaces, temperature and scents of what you are eating can assist with segment control. Yet, mindful eating additionally implies securing on the thing you are eating and when — this can assist you with recognizing needless chomping minutes you may not understand you are taking part in for the day that might be steering on excess calories. Even more importantly, make an effort to abstain from consuming food sources that you haven't chosen for yourself. Eating mindfully can help you shift the focus of control from external experts and signals to your body's wisdom. Understanding the source of your repeated calories is another step in making better decisions in the short and long term.

6. Enliven your life.

Shocking food sources can assist you with scaling back calories. That is because capsaicin, an emulsion set up in jalapeño and cayenne peppers, may(marginally) increase your body's arrival of stress chemicals like adrenaline, which can accelerate your capacity to consume calories. What is further, eating hot peppers might help you eat all the more languidly and keep away from ravenousness. You are bound to remain more mindful of when you are full. A few extraordinary decisions other than hot peppers are energy and turmeric.

7. Hit the sack previously.

There is a lot of investigation that shows getting lower than they got some information about seven hours — of rest each night can decelerate your digestion. Constant rest privation may for sure modify chemicals that control craving, and a few examinations show that there's an association between low-quality decisions and lower rest. Great rest has a lot of different advantages as well, such as supporting readiness, culminating state of mind and generally speaking personal satisfaction. So don't ration your ZZZs, and you will be granted an excess edge with regards to generally speaking well-being and getting fitter. Fire a little simply by moving up sleep time by 15 to 30 sparkles, each nanosecond counts!

8. Keep a food diary.

Individuals who log all that they eat — particularly the people who log while they are eating — are bound to get in shape and keep it off for the long stretch, concentrating continually demonstrating. The propensity likewise takes lower than 15 sparkles each day on normal when you do it routinely, as per a review distributed in the diary Heftiness.

Begin following an application like MyFitnessPal or utilize a standard tablet. It will assist you with remaining liable for what you've eaten. Furthermore, you can smoothly distinguish regions that could utilize a little upgrade when it's worked out before you.

9. Repulse the craving to skirt a wreck.
Our sustenance specialists stress that skipping reflections won't cause you to shed pounds quickly. Nonetheless, store a piece of products of the soil of nut worship in your auto or pack and keep snacks in your office opening — anything that will hold you back from going void!
If an energized day makes a plunk-down wreck insolvable.
Going long periods without food performs a twofold responsibility disadvantage on our good dieting sweats by both decelerating your digestion and preparing you for a gorge hitherto in the day. Make it your charge to eat three reflections and two snacks consistently, and don't remain longer than three to four hours without eating. Set a" nibble caution" on your telephone whenever requested.

10. Chomp on mineral-rich food varieties.

Potassium, magnesium and calcium can assist with filling in as an external equilibrium for bulge changing over sodium. Food varieties that are wealthy in potassium incorporate verdant vegetation, the most extreme" orange" food varieties(oranges, yams, carrots, melon), bananas, tomatoes, and cruciferous veggies, particularly cauliflower. Nuts, seeds, low-fat dairy, and low-fat dairy products can all help you reduce swelling. They have also been linked to a wide range of novel medicinal benefits, including lowering blood pressure, managing glucose, and generally lowering the risk of common complaints.

CHAPTER THREE

TIME-BOUND EATING

Time-bound eating is an eating routine securing on wreck timing as opposed to calorie input. An individual on a period-restricted eating(TRE) plan will just eat during explicit hours and will gormandize at any remaining times.

In this section, we take a gander at what TRE is, whether it works, and what impact it has on muscle gain.

We additionally give first-year recruits tips on th,e best way to begin with this eating plan.

What's time-restricted eating?

TRE implies that an individual eats their appearance in general and snacks inside a specific window of time every day. This time can fluctuate as indicated by the individual's inclination and the arrangement they decide to follow. By and large, in any case, the eating window in time-restricted programs goes from 6 - 12 hours every day.

Beyond this period, an individual consumes no calories. They might hydrate or have no-calorie beverages to remain splashed. In some TRE plans, individuals may likewise consume slender espresso or tea with no cream.

TRE is a kind of discontinuous fasting. This alludes to any eating plan that shifts back and forth between times restricting calories and eating regularly.

Although TRE won't work for everybody, some might think that it is healthy. Ongoing examinations have demonstrated the way that it can promote weight reduction and may bring down the danger of metabolic circumstances, like diabetes.
Without tracking calories, TRE might help someone cut back on their food intake. Additionally, it can be a good approach to avoid common food risks like late-night snacking. In any case, those with diabetes or other health issues should consider speaking with a croaker before undertaking this type of dietary strategy.

Does it work for weight reduction?

There isn't a single diet that will help everyone lose weight. While some people will certainly achieve the weight loss goals associated with TRE, others might not. A person should consult a croaker before attempting TRE or any other dietary regimen.

Ongoing examinations affecting individuals of various periods and in various investigation settings show that TRE has the verifiable to prompt weight reduction and well-being upgrade:

> **Weight reduction:** As per 21 randomized controlled preliminary in Nourishment and Diabetes, 30 guys and women with portliness who followed two months of TRE with an attractive get-healthy plan saw a clinically significant weight reduction of about 24 pounds(lb) on ordinary, contrasted and around 20 lb in the 30 individuals not doing TRE.
>
> **Metabolic example and heart grumbling:** A recent report in the Diary of Translational Medication set up that 20 women with portliness who followed TRE for a considerable length of time lost generally 7.5

lb on normal from their beginning review weight. The TRE group also improved risk variables for both cardiac protests and metabolic problems.

Stomach microbiome: According to a recent investigation, about 9 lb of weight was lost overall in a group of 25 obese people who followed TRE for a very long period, along with minor changes to the stomach microbiota's appearance. The experimenters observed that these progressions' clinical significance is still unclear.

Organism synthesis: In a recent article published in Wildernesses in Sustenance, clinical and real data from 43 randomized controlled preliminary studies with 2,438 review participants aged 18 to 79 were analyzed. Discontinuous fasting, including TRE, led to increased weight loss and alterations in body composition when compared to non-mediation schedules.

Type 2 diabetes: For the activity of type 2 diabetes, a 2022 survey in The Diary of Physiology set up that TRE offers the advantage of gentle weight reduction and better glucose activity.

Some investigation takes note that medical advantages might be valid on the off chance that individuals don't shed pounds because of attempting TRE.

Cell digestion has distributed one of the most rigorously directed randomized controlled preliminaries to date. It set up that when eight guys with prediabetes who were fat followed early TRE for quite some time, a few marks of heart well-being were bettered, including:

- insulin perceptivity
- the ability of the pancreatic cells responsible for producing insulin to withstand oxidative stress

When the TRE group didn't become in shape and displayed a lesser desire to eat at night, changes in heart health were evident. To confirm these findings, researchers need to conduct additional tests over longer periods on more subjects.

Is it preferred for weight reduction over standard calorie limitation?

Collecting investigation recommends that TRE has understood, however, not all reviews show it's further powerful for weight reduction than diurnal standard calorie limitation.

A 2017 survey inferred that discontinuous calorie limitation, including TRE, offers no critical benefit over restricting calorie input every day.

All the more of late, a 2022 randomized controlled clinical preliminary in the New Britain Diary of Medication showed TRE had no weight reduction benefit following a year.

In the preliminary, 139 individuals with heftiness followed TRE while additionally eating more modest calories or following diurnal calorie limitation alone. At the point when the review finished, there were no distinctions between the gatherings for weight reduction.

Studies from 2019 and 2022 note that TRE brings about equivalent weight reduction to normal diurnal calorie limitation in individuals who are fat or have heftiness.

Along these lines, TRE can be a possibility for individuals who need a substitute outcome to diurnal calorie limitation for weight reduction.

Other investigation shows no advantage of TRE for weight reduction contrasted and eating consistently over the day with no calorie limitation. This incorporates when concentrating on entertainers conceding no guidance to change their food decisions or effort circumstances.

As the insight on TRE for weight reduction progresses, a few experimenters have communicated the requirement for an alert around who should seriously mull over following TRE.

Among individuals who are fat or have stoutness, a few examinations have set up that weight reduction in TRE might be because of the deficiency of extra mass(muscle) versus fat mass(fat towel).

In this manner, it's particularly significant for individuals who are fat or have heftiness and who likewise have comorbidities like sarcopenia to chat with a croaker before attempting TRE.

Does TRE work for long-haul weight preservation?

The ongoing validation base shows a vow for the piece of TRE in weight reduction temporarily(from concentrates on enduring lower than a half year).

In any case, experimenters need longer-term studies with bigger figures of additional various entertainers to decide if TRE can prompt clinically significant weight reduction that an individual can keep up with over the long run.

A recent report from the diary Craving intended to check out at the walls or facilitators of following TRE over the long haul. It utilized 20 moderately aged adults who were fat or had portliness and were in danger of type 2 diabetes.

The experimenters surveyed how smoothly individuals could integrate TRE into diurnal life following a 3-month study with organized interviews.

Seven review entertainers stayed aware of their directions on TRE from the review, 10 accustomed their way to dealing with following an alternate understanding of their unique guidelines, and three didn't adhere to their guidelines.

Difficulties in staying aware of TRE in the long haul included:

- eating ethics while going to get-togethers
- conflicting timetables of diurnal life
- unpredictable eating events
- not gathering weight reduction assumptions
- the nonappearance of family support
- interests of responsibility or tone-fault

Experimenters need further work to comprehend what TRE means for the normal, social, psychosocial, and ecological facilitators of and walls to effective long-haul weight protection.

Keeping up with muscle and TRE

The investigation has shown that TRE doesn't feel to influence the general protection of muscle adversely. In a 2019 study, TRE was investigated in 11 obese persons. They followed the early TRE schedule for four days, eating from 8 a.m. to 2 p.m., before switching to the control schedule, which calls for eating from 8 a.m. to 8 p.m.

The authors concluded that when performers implemented the early-TRE plan, mTOR effort was increased. This protein marker is approved to be used in maintaining bulk.

A recent report, in the American Diary of Clinical Sustenance, randomly doled out 16 else solid guys to follow early-TRE for quite some time or simply standard calorie limitation. It set up the TRE bunch and saw a better capacity for their muscle to utilize glucose and fanned-chain amino acids.

A recent report in Logical Reports doled out 46 else solid matured guys to follow a month and a half of either TRE or their normal eating plan. The TRE bunch had no huge changes in their bulk. This proposes the entertainers kept their muscles all through the review period.

In examinations that matched TRE with an organized obstruction preparing program, the bulk was kept up with or little profit in muscle well-being happened:

> **Muscle development:** A recent report randomly relegated 40 otherwise sound and dynamic energetic women to about two months of following their standard eating design, TRE, or TRE and a helpful enhancement with a connection to muscle

upgrade. Muscle execution and muscle development improved with no significant contrasts between the gatherings.

Protection of extra mass and muscle strength: A recent report set up that a month of TRE and a 25% decrease in calories kept spare mass similarly situated as a normal calorie limitation in 26 dynamic energetic guys. The two gatherings saw an equivalent misfortune in muscle-to-fat ratio without unfavourable products on their extra mass or muscle strength.

Muscle abidance: A recent report erratically relegated 21 moderately aged adults who were fat or had stoutness to finish two months of TRE or standard eating for quite some time. The two gatherings had a little expansion in spare mass, muscle strength, and muscle abidance.

Muscle Execution and protein input: A recent report requested that 20 energetic guys stay with their TRE or standard eating design for 10 excess months. As indicated by the 2021 review that distributed the outcomes, the two gatherings expanded their seat press and leg press execution despite losing without fat mass. The TRE group maintained a protein intake of 1.9 grams per kilogram of body weight while maintaining a 10-energy decline.

The summation of validation recommends that in blend with opposition preparation, TRE might enhance body synthesis and assist individuals with keeping up with sans fat mass likewise to non-TRE plans. Without fat mass incorporates the body's muscles, organs, bones, and water content.

A few experimenters note that TRE may not be the a la mode approach assuming essential well-being assumptions incorporate raising bulk and consummating muscle strength due to the conflicting eating recurrence and supplement vacuity for muscles.
In any case, TRE might be a decent volition for certain individuals who are keen on changing their body structure or shedding pounds without it being dangerous for keeping up with bulk, development, strength, execution, or abidance.

Experimenters need new longer and bigger examinations in various investigation settings with various populaces to grasp the connection between TRE and muscle wellbeing.

An individual ought to consider talking with a croaker about the' merchandise TRE might have on muscle wellbeing.

Beginning with time-confined eating

One of TRE's key advantages is that no unique feasts or apparatuses are required. An individual can begin a TRE plan immediately after securing a specialist's OK.

To improve the probability of progress, as with any dietary routine, some thought and arranging are important. TRE might be made to be more secure and more effective by utilizing the accompanying exhortation:

Beginning gradually

Starting with a more limited fasting period, individuals ought to stretch it bit by bit over the long run. Begin your quick, for example, from 10:00 p.m. until 6:30 a.m. To get to the objective fasting time frame, then, at that point, increment this by 30 minutes like clockwork.

Studies have proposed that binding taking care of ages to lower than 6 hours is dicey to offer new benefits over additional drawn-out taking care of ages.

Practising without exaggerating it

It's enticing to begin an incredible activity plan close by eating lower for quicker results. In any case, with TRE, this can make the fasting time frame more sensitive.

Individuals might wish to keep their exercise program something similar until their body changes with the new eating plan. This can assist with keeping away from expanded hunger from excess activities, which might conceive breakdown or disappointment.

Securing on protein and fibre

Appetite can be sensitive for individuals who don't have experience fasting for a few hours every day. Picking food varieties wealthy in fibre and protein during the eating window can assist with combatting this. These supplements help an individual vibe full and can assist blood with the sugaring crash or food jones.

For outline, an individual might eat entire grain toss and pasta as opposed to white or refined grains.

They can pick a bite that remembers protein for the type of extra meat, egg, tofu, or nuts.

Trying not to object to slips

Having days where TRE doesn't work out is ordinary. For representation, a night out with musketeers, a unique event, or an oversight might prompt individuals to eat beyond their proper eating window.

In any case, this doesn't imply that they ought to stop.

It's in vogue to consider slips to be an event to refocus. On an approaching day, individuals can recommence the TRE plan and go on toward their thing.

Focus Point

For most extreme individuals, TRE is suspected to be a peculiar weight reduction fix. In any case, studies have demonstrated the way that it can offer medical advantages without a high danger of side merchandise.

It tends to be a basic way for various individuals to diminish their calorie input without confounded or severe eating routine standards.

CHAPTER FOUR

GOOD FOOD DRUTHERS TO GET THINNER

Shedding pounds can be tiring, yet integrating quality food druthers can have a tremendous effect. Pick zoodles as opposed to surveys, close for avocado instead of worship, favour hummus over mayo, and change to contributed water as opposed to soft drink. Consider protein balls as a cover for delicacy bars, pick trail mix over chips, and close with quinoa over rice. Frozen yoghurt is a better volition than frozen yoghurt. For available and dietary choices, investigate the Clean Eatz Kitchen wreck plans, which incorporate a weight reduction wreck plan conveyed right to your doorstep. Begin rolling out sure improvements with these good food varieties to get in shape and enhance your general well-being.

Zoodles over Noodles

Zoodles are a dietary and waist cordial choice to conventional surveys, drafted from zucchini. These veggie gyrations have earned colossal elegance, without a doubt advancing into the frozen food path of your unique supermarket. Loaded with fundamental supplements, cell reinforcements, more than adequate hydration, and fibre, finishing up for zoodles as opposed to surveys can offer plenty of well-being tips. These benefits envelop glucose guidelines, upgraded absorption, advanced cardiovascular prosperity, and assisted weight reduction preliminaries. When joined with a variety of new vegetables, zoodles can act as the establishment for an elegant processing plant-grounded pasta cover wreck.

Avocado over Butter

Jump into any well-being food diner and you're certain to track down avocado toast on their menu! Be that as it may, for what reason is it so famous? Avocado is one the very pinnacle supplement of thick food sources you can find and is thought of as a" superfood" due to being loaded with fibre, folate, potassium, Vitamin E, magnesium, Vitamin B6, and L-ascorbic acid. Moreover, this mutable organic product is stacked with Omega-3s, which are one of the ideal solid fats to remember for the eating regimen. The medical advantages of remembering avocado for the eating regimen remember decreases in cholesterol, progressions in heart wellbeing, improvement of exemption, decreases in joint pain or exercise-persuaded aggravation, and upgrades in skin wellbeing. Since avocado is a processing plant grounded fat, changing it out with hero worship implies the end of impregnated fats. So where could you at any point view an avocado on the run? Search for good food druthers that advance weight reduction and back your prosperity. Avocado is a high delineation of one of these quality food varieties to get thinner while partaking in a delicious wreck.

Hummus over Mayo

What's hummus produced using and how can it connect with weight reduction? This good food volition is a glue produced using ground chickpeas, olive oil painting, sesame, and various flavours. Ounce for ounce, you'll find 75 more modest calories in hummus contrasted with mayo! In any case, it isn't just about the calories. Hummus likewise contains a blend of nutrients and minerals, with the main ones being calcium, folate, zinc, B-Nutrients, and Vitamin E. This blend of supplements adds to headways in bone well-being, energy circumstances, and weak capability. With around 8 grams of processing plant-grounded protein per serving, you get to partake in some muscle-structure benefits while staying away from the impregnated fat set up in mayo, which advances heart well-being. The low glycemic marker and high fibre content of hummus assist with overseeing glucose while supporting ideal processing. Since one of the principal constituents is an olive oil painting, this one-of-a-kind good food volition likewise advances diminished irritation.

Imbued Water over Soda

Did you have at least some idea that there are about 17 scoops of sugar in a 20-oz customary soft drink? Likewise, a jug of customary soft drink can contain as significant as 250 kcal! This is generally unique to the volume of a common inexpensive food drink, disregarding the free restorations that various individuals exploit. Cering this it's assessed that it takes 3500 kcal to acquire or lose one pound of muscle versus fat. What's the significance here of your alarming statement about weight gain? Polishing off customary soft drinks or tacky beverages two or three times each day for seven days gets you positioned to acquire a pound consistently! That is 4 lbs each month and 48 lbs every time! That's what the positive news is assuming you're a soft drink clincher, you can likewise advance weight reduction at a similar rate by banishing it from your eating regimen. A simple and savvy volition contributed to water. Water contributed with foods grown from the ground offers endless understood benefits, including upgrading digestion, advancing skin wellbeing, abetting in weight activity, directing pulse, consummating absorption, improving nutrient submersion, helping weak wellbeing, facilitating exercise recuperation, and supporting mental capability.

Protein Balls over Sweet treats

Can we just be real for a moment? We as a whole need a sugar fix, and delicacy is by all accounts all over — managing machines, service stations, and snack bars. Sooner or later, we are probably going to enjoy a delicacy to fulfil our sweet Jones, except if we plan ahead of time. In any case, extra-large delicacy bars, stacked with north of 500 kcal, can cause obliteration for a weight activity wreck plan. Taking into account that it just takes an overabundance of 3500 kcal to acquire one pound of muscle versus fat, it's scary how snappily this can be with calorie-thick delicacy bars! Tragically, these delicacy bars offer the least nutritive worth past calories. As a better volition, you can create protein balls that mirror the sweet and flavorful blend set up in delicacy bars while boosting nutritive substance. As opposed to commonly added sugars, protein balls compute on dried organic products, honey, and little amounts of sweet treats. Protein can be pressed in with nut hero worship, blended nuts, and protein maquillages. In addition, mitigating constituents like flaxseed, chia seeds, and hemp hearts can be consolidated.

Trail Blend over Chips

Chips are a famous nibble for various people since they're promptly accessible, bear no refrigeration, and can be consumed in a hurry. In any case, chips regularly contain high amounts of impregnated fat and sodium, the two of which aren't great for heart well-being or weight activity. Likewise, chips are restricted to each flavour and surface in turn, prompting thoughtless utilization and restricted fulfilment. Trail blends offer a fabulous volition to chips, permitting us to plan them for expanded fulfilment and better nutritive worth decisively. While securing on weight activity, the ideal starting point for a path mix is low-sodium popcorn, which is low in calories and gives the asked crunch undifferentiated from chips. The constituents we add to upgrade the mix help our fulfilment. A mix of sweet, pungent, delicate, and brickle variables has been demonstrated to generally fulfil. Consider consolidating points of interest like dried organic products, nuts, seeds, an extra protein like hamburger jerky, and little partitions of liberal deals with dim chocolate.

Quinoa over Rice

To be sure assuming you are weird with it, quinoa(sharp · waa) is a great rice volition! While they've undifferentiated in calorie content, quinoa outperforms rice concerning nourishment. Initially, quinoa is viewed as a total protein source, containing every one of the nine fundamental amino acids, very much like customary eat-grounded proteins. Quinoa's protein content is almost twofold that of rice. Fibre and carb circumstances are comparative among quinoa and rice, so there is no concession in these perspectives while doing the switch. In general, quinoa offers 3-4 times the supplement content of earthy-coloured rice, including bountiful amounts of iron, manganese, phosphorus, magnesium, zinc, calcium, potassium, and selenium.

Frozen Yogurt over Ice Cream

It's inarguable that frozen yoghurt is a well-known treat! all things considered, various of us come worried about our weight when we enjoy excessively significant weight. A viable outcome is to substitute customary frozen yoghurt with frozen yoghurt, which essentially diminishes calories and fat contribution while possibly adding protein content by 5-6 times! As opposed to depending on locally acquired frozen yoghurt, I suggest that my visitors mix vanilla Greek yoghurt with their lean toward foods grown from the ground. This outcome in a high-protein" snowstorm" without extreme fat and calories. For those looking for additional inventiveness, you can indurate the Greek yoghurt blend into popsicles.

Focus point

All in all, consolidating quality food druthers can have a massive effect on weight reduction sweats and general well-being. By simplifying trades, like picking zoodles over surveys, avocado over applause, hummus over mayo, and contributed water over soft drink, you can appreciate delicious reflections while decreasing calorie and fat info. Protein balls can act as a wonderful cover for delicacy bars, while trail mix offers a more healthful choice contrasted with chips. Quinoa gives a supplement-rich volition to rice, and solidified yoghurt is a better decision than customary frozen yoghurt. In addition, investigating wreck plans like the Clean Eatz Kitchen can offer available and wholesome choices for weight reduction. Begin rolling out sure improvements with these quality food sources to get thinner and enhance your general well-being.

CHAPTER FIVE

THE DIFFICULTIES IN DELAYED FASTING

Fasting, the deliberate limitation of calorie input throughout some time, has incalculable medical advantages including weight reduction, assurance against grumblings and better life. It comes in various structures, the most famous for weight reduction being hauled (enduring longer than two days) and discontinuous(scattering between patterns of fasting and devouring). The two styles enjoy various benefits and inconveniences relying upon your life - however which is better for weight reduction?

How does fasting function?
Sweet limitation advances weight reduction through the course of ketosis, during which the body processes fat for energy. Around 12-16 hours into voila, blood glucose and insulin circumstances drop and the supplement flagging pathways that are controlled by the mTOR kinase protein are killed.

This powers the body into the fasting state and it begins to change from involving glucose from nourishment for energy to using fat stores, creating ketones that are oxidized by the mind. As food is welcomed, supplement flagging pathways are reactivated and ketosis plateaus. This cycle can advance weight reduction as well as improve metabolic capability, decrease aggravation and upgrade weak working. Weight reduction has countless advantages to well-being and life, diminishing the danger of bleakness from heart objections, stroke, type 2 diabetes and a few tumours.

Ketosis enjoys the new benefit of consuming fat inventories without utilizing protein, making it conceivable to proceed with weight lifting for keeping up with and developing muscle during sweet limitation.

What's hauled fasting?
The human body has accustomed to repulsing long times of food privation, with the longest quick at any point recorded enduring 382 days.

Hauled fasting is an outrageous type of sweet limitation that goes on for two days or further. For the most part, they last anywhere between 2-5 days to about fourteen days and are just broken by the utilization of water and plain tea or espresso. For those new to fasting, it's suggested that you practice irregular diets of adding lengths before attempting hauled, as your body becomes adjusted to ketosis.

For outline, begin with the 12:12 discontinuous presto before continuing toward a 24-hour quick and at last a two-day hauled voila.

Advantages to well-being and life

Hauled fasting can advance weight reduction, decrease stomach fat and enhance pulse circumstances, without a doubt in people who are previously a sound weight.

It's anything but a fast weight reduction fix and ought to be rehashed routinely, for outline one time each month, to see the actual consequences of long-haul weight reduction. Hauled enjoys an upper hand over short discontinuous diets in that it actuates autophagy, the course of cell revivification. Autophagy is a continuous cell process in which cells practice their harmed organelles to restore.

It's likewise utilized during supplement pressure to adjust accessible energy hotspots for endurance and accordingly can be ignited by sweet limitation. Close to 24 hours into a hauled voila, supplement seeing pathways stifle the Slope kinase protein in light of supplement privation, changing over autophagy.

The cell reestablishment from autophagy is taken into account overage-related grievances like neurodegeneration, cardiomyopathy, and diabetes and can abide as an increment in life. Autophagy arrives at its loftiest situation around day two of a hauled voila, so is more sensitive to accomplish utilizing more limited irregular quick styles.

Implied Side Products

A heinous charge to hauled fasting is the steady yearning that goes with supported calorie limitation. Taking into account that most extreme delayed diets just permit the utilization of water, tea and espresso, a framework requires serious responsibility and incitement. In any case, our bodies can adjust to cravings and one review set up that 93% of subjects revealed a shortfall of appetite.

While hauled fasting is for the most part protected, it's one of the dangerous styles of sweet limitation that can be joined by gentle side products including dehumidification, electrolyte lopsidedness and exhaustion. junkies additionally may observe backwardness and low energy as the body advances into ketosis. This can be battled by going to reasonable lengths like adding your water input, adding ½-1 tablespoon of sea swab to drinking water to help electrolyte decrease, and taking ordinary rest.

An essential sort of hauled presto is the fasting-mirroring diet, a five-a-day presto that gives supplements an extraordinarily planned wreck plan without driving the body's supplement seeing pathways and keeping up with the fasting state. This is a more straightforward choice for individuals who need to attempt hauled fasting while at the same time keeping away from the feared hunger that accompanies customary diets.

CHAPTER SIX

THE TRANSIENT STYLE OF LIFE

Discontinuous fasting is what?
Doubtlessly, you've heard some persuasive achievement stories concerning discontinuous fasting. Nonetheless, is fasting solid, and is it compelling to be irregularly quick?

A customary practice that is innocuous when not exaggerated is fasting, which includes halting eating for some time. Fasting has forever been related to otherworldly and substantial benefits. Fasting for strict objects is often connected with a more prominent focus on otherworldly issues. Truly, a concise quick bring down glucose brings down irritation helps digestion, flushes poisons from harmed cells, and has been related to diminished malignant growth risk, further ligament eruptions, and worked on mental capability.

Discontinuous fasting is the act of routinely switching back and forth between "eating windows" and times of forbearance. A normal irregular fasting plan would forbid eating between the long periods of 7:00 a.m. also, 3:00 p.m. also, command fasting for the other 16 hours of the day. In any case, there is no set, framed plan. Certain individuals set higher or less indulgent eating limitations, for example, not eating after 8:00 p.m., or, on the altogether less permissive finish of the range, just allowing themselves to eat every other day.

Discontinuous fasting's science is centred around adjusting the body's digestion. Without nourishment for some time, insulin levels tumble to where the body begins consuming fat for energy. Also, it is accepted that by easing back the body's digestion, you would decrease your craving and eat less when you continue eating.

The benefits of irregular fasting for weight reduction have been displayed in various examinations. It's muddled at this point whether it works any better compared to simply caloric limitation and customary dietary patterns. The viability of irregular fasting might be expected to some degree to the way that most experts have surrendered the act of eating late night and night. Eating just in the first part of the day is more on top of our circadian rhythms and less inclined to bring about food being put away as fat. A reasonable substitute for discontinuous fasting might be to consume a low-calorie Mediterranean eating routine and to wrap up eating them in the late evening because numerous people find it challenging to adhere to it.

Certain individuals, like those with diabetes or coronary illness, shouldn't endeavour irregular fasting without first counselling their PCP.

Since discontinuous fasting is such a "way of life escalated" dietary procedure, it tends to be hard to support amid standard sauvignons. You could be enticed to break your quick if the remainder of your family is eating while you're not or to quit having family feasts by and large. You'll find it trying to keep up an irregular fasting plan assuming your work constrains you to have feasts with clients or collaborators. Remember that the good dieting plan you will adhere to is the best one.

Well-known fasting of this sort requests less devotion than long-haul fasting. It involves switching back and forth between eating and fasting stretches, either inside a solitary day or north of a few days and can in some cases be ceaseless. The way that it doesn't limit what you eat during devouring periods recognizes it from a traditional eating routine. Substitute day fasting, and substitute and the one dinner daily quick (OMAD) are a couple of instances of the different discontinuous fasting designs.

Time-limited eating (TRE) likewise shifts back and forth between fasting and eating times inside a solitary day, for example, the 12:12, 16:8, and more thorough 20:4. Everybody takes part in TRE somewhat while they rest, consequently drawing out this compulsory quick is a straightforward way to deal with incorporating TRE into a lifestyle.

Benefits For Wellbeing

Indeed, even the most limited discontinuous diets can bring about similar fat-copying impacts of delayed fasting since ketosis begins to happen 12 to 16 hours quickly.

In contrast with extended fasting, irregular fasting enjoys the benefit of not causing outrageous food cravings and should be possible consistently. This brings down the quick's adverse consequences on different parts of life, such as mingling, and makes it more straightforward to adhere to. Integrating them can assist you restore your relationship with food. Clients have revealed encountering less craving, an alternate reaction to eating, and worked on prosperity.

Notwithstanding, with constrained extended diets, it turns out to be more difficult to encounter autophagy's cell restoration benefits with brief discontinuous diets since it begins no less than 16 hours into a quick, contingent upon the person.

Conceivable Adverse Consequences

Contrasted with delayed fasting, discontinuous fasting conveys less risk and has fewer secondary effects like freezing and weakness. To compensate for the calorie limitation, a few people, notwithstanding, may unexpectedly diminish their actual work and increment their energy consumption previously, during, and after a period of fasting, reducing the benefits of the quick.

Trying not to gorge and taking part in humble action, which isn't exhorted during delayed diets, are two methods for halting this. Both irregular and broadened fasting are successful weight reduction procedures, and keeping in mind that drawn-out fasting enjoys the additional benefit of advancing autophagy, discontinuous fasting is a less complex option for long-haul weight reduction because of its serious calorie limitation.

CHAPTER SEVEN

NORMAL DETERRENTS

Whether you might want to drop five pounds or 50, it can feel like there are 1,000,000 weight reduction impediments hindering you.

Getting fitter is generally difficult, and there may be various inner, calculated, and life elements to defeat to arrive at your thing.

Be that as it may, don't surrender. You can shed those obstinate pounds with just enough soul-looking (Do I disdain cauliflower?) and a few pragmatic tips(remain, I can revitalize cauliflower?? This is SO Great!).

To augment your odds of coming out on top, begin by taking many sparkles to distinguish your greatest hindrances to getting in shape and perceive how you can beat them.

They are 12 of the most widely recognized bones that hinder shedding pounds:

Diet Deterrents

1. Handicap You lack the opportunity and energy to cook.
Result: Accomplish some fixed work.
Nobody is denying it's more straightforward to arrange takeout than it's to make a ware from scratch. Be that as it may, cooking solid reflections doesn't need to be a significant time-suck.
A few scrumptious choices — like a primary course salad — to be sure bear no cooking by any means. The key is to assume what you'll eat sometime before your breadbasket begins snarling.

Dietitian Tammy Lakatos Disgrace, R.D.N., CFT, co-creator of The Nourishment Twins' Veggie Fix, suggests setting aside time at the end of the week to plan your outfits for the following week, stock up on ingredients, and prepare specific vegetables and protein so you'll look great when you peer into the ice chest after a challenging day at work.

2. Handicap You despise being vacant.
Result: Bring about freight over on low-calorie, filling food sources.
Shock You don't need to eat bitsy amounts of food to get in shape. You're in an ideal situation not denying yourself or you could wind up falling enough snappily.

According to Lakatos Disgrace, "the sharp way for feeling full—and being slimmer is to top off with a quintet of whole grains, foods cultivated from the ground, and extra protein. In the absence of protein and fibre to slow down digestion, "(Reused or basic) Carbs by themselves will give you energy, but you'll crash soon after."

She's additionally dependent on keeping bunches of non-boring veggies available, similar to broccoli, Brussels fledglings, cauliflower, and squash.

"To spice up excellent beans, add marmalade. On the other hand, she suggests stirring them up so they caramelize and taste delicious.

In addition to the fact that they are loaded up with heaps of nourishment(nutrients, minerals, and phytonutrients), the fibre and water will assist with topping you off.

3. Handicap You could do without the flavour of quality food.

Result: Be patient and continue to attempt new impacts.

You, most importantly, may not understand what great, healthful food poses a flavour like. (Suggest It's not straight, bland funk and limp, overcooked veggies.)

Watch a solid cooking show to become familiar with the essentials and preliminary for certain new moulds. Need a few thoughts? You can find a large number of choices right then.

In any case, if you simply assume nothing will taste great except if it's pan-fried and stacked with swabs or sugar, show restraint.

As you make out your structure power and attempt new impacts, you'll find food sources you appreciate, and for sure bones that don't feel enchanting right presently could at last come to your pets.

4. Handicap You guess dietary food is excessively valuable.

Result: Go with brilliant decisions.

Spendy natural yield is perfect, however, it's not fundamental for good well-being or weight reduction, says Lakatos Disgraces.

Attempt to look for what's in-season — it's almost consistently less expensive and streaks back that frozen vegetables and natural products are by and large as wholesome as their new partners.

Lakatos Disgraces likewise prompts her visitors who are on a careful spending plan to eat further compliant and industrial facility-grounded protein while restricting valuable points of interest, similar to meat.

Furthermore, assuming you guess that voila food quintet wreck is less expensive than a solid serving of mixed greens, assume once more.

Investigation proposes that remaining fit and solid could save you difficult money in well-being-related pursuits on the street.

Furthermore, without a doubt temporarily, getting fitter can be bring-powerful if you believe it should be, says Holly Lucille, N.D., R.N., a Los Angeles-grounded naturopathic croaker and CrossFit mentor. She claims that drinking less wine and cutting out on socializing outings are effective ways to save some magnates.

Wellness Deterrents

5. Handicap You guess practice is exhausting.
Result: Find the item you love.
In any case, likewise, you're doing some unacceptable drill If you think about your drill as a task. Risking a pleasant effort is urgent if you have any desire to stay with it long enough to get in shape and keep it off.

All things considered, don't do it. On the off chance that running a routine is similarly instigative to you as expanding at an oversight wall.

Preliminary with different sorts of activities until you find a solid match Attempt a nation-line moving class, fight some butt in a blended military exchanges drill, or look at a yoga class; your choices are perpetual!

Furthermore, if you're simply trying things out, the sleek spot to begin is at the morning 21-Day Fix with Pre-winter Calabrese is an extraordinary method for fighting beginning your excursion.

6. Handicap You lack the opportunity and willpower to work out.
Result: Track down a drill that accommodates your timetable.

Absence of time is quite possibly the greatest wall, but on the other hand, it's tied in with making practices a priority, says Lakatos Disgraces. Recording an opportunity in your day like you would an arrangement can assist you with doing that.

Be that as it may, if you're time-lashed, ensure you're taking advantage of your perspiration meetings. Pick a drill that is intended to snappily yield significant outcomes.

Shaun T's Change 20 and Occupation 1 with Jennifer Jacobs, for delineation, were made to get you an hour of results in less than 30 minutes.

The two projects likewise utilize extreme cardio exercise(HIIT), which assists you with consuming further calories each nanosecond contrasted with a consistent state workout.

You likewise continue to consume further calories for quite a long time in this way.

By shifting your power position, you lower your heart rate repeatedly, increase post-practice oxygen consumption, and end up burning calories after your drill is ended, according to Lucille.

Or on the other hand, if you're an early riser, Morning Complete Implosion 100 with Jericho McMatthews highlights 100 one-of-a-kind 20-to-30-nanosecond works out.

7. Handicap You propel yourself excessively hard, too often.

Result: Make recuperation a priority.

Strolling your canine around the block might get your heart siphoning somewhat, yet it's rarely sufficient to assist you with shedding pounds.

Moreover, it's not difficult to overdo it, and certain individuals wind up hitting wellness plateaus since they never give their bodies the time they need to recuperate from each of the savage activities they're doing.

It's crucial to give yourself enough time to recover, advises Lucille. My speed and viability improve when I have to take a little break and go back to the spa.

Yet, before you get excessively fomented, " recuperation " doesn't approach " lying on the settee the entire day with the remote. "

There's a distinction between rest and recuperation days; on rest days, you'll need to focus on getting rest and recharging your energy stores.

On recuperation days, you can in any case work out, however to a lower degree. Attempt a delicate yoga routine from multi Week Yoga Retreat or these full-body extensions.

The statement made by Lucille was that "your body needs to be tested by doing something it's not used to."

8. Handicap You work out activities to do everything.

Result: Comprehend that exercise is simply an aspect of the perplexity.

While exercise can most likely assist you with getting in shape, you can't expect results assuming that you focus on wellness while overlooking terrible dietary patterns.

Investigation shows that individuals who start a solid eating routine AND a drill program simultaneously are bound to recently be doing both a period.

Approximately 60% of weight loss is due to diet, and 40% is due to exercise, according to Lucille.

In any case, sustenance programs like Part Fix and 2B Mentality can teach you(and your family!) to make good dieting a day-to-day existence, If you don't know where to begin.

9. Handicap Your joints torment.
Result: Go low-influence.

Whether you're recuperating from a physical issue or have an ongoing issue, it's difficult to move when you're in torment.

Expecting you have your croaker's alright, take a stab at moving forward your effort a tiny bit of touch, and focus on low-influence work out, says Lakatos Disgraces.

" Any development at each is superior to sitting on the settee, and without a doubt burning through 30 sparkles on an activity bicycle or swimming might assist you with getting thinner if you were sufficiently stationary previously, " she makes sense of.

Profound Snags

10. Handicap You're simply not excessively spurred.

Result: Set short and long-haul assumptions.

There's a justification for why getting fitter before a marriage or institute reunion is as often as possible simpler.

However, inspirations like that will more often than not be temporary, and in practically no time, those 10 pounds(or further) are back on.

Setting a long-term,non-scale thing - — say, to stay away from medical problems that a parent or grandparent has — will help, yet you'll probably require a few excess focuses to go for en route.

I once significantly reduced my weight by pushing myself to perform a certain number of drive-ups every day until I could perform 100, recalls Lucille.

Certain individuals find that getting cutthroat — perhaps by buying into a progression of overwhelming occasions, similar to a half-long distance race or 5K — keeps them putting resources into remaining fit.

11. Handicap You're humiliated by your bombed endeavours.

Result: Let it go, reconsider, and reboot.

Bunches of individuals attempt to get thinner and continually fall flat, and they wind up whipping themselves.

In any case, Lucille recommends nixing disgrace and fault by doing a 21-day " necropsy " — go through five sparkles every late evening evaluating your propensities and permitting about what went right(and what didn't) that day, and make an effort not to make any brutal decisions, Assuming that sounds like you.

The thing is to eventually have an " aha " second that empowers you to quit feeling shamefaced and rather permits you to focus on pushing ahead.

12.   Handicap   Your   restriction   vanishes notwithstanding enticement.

Result: Bring about arranging your safeguard.

At times it could feel like the whole world is on a mission to undermine your weight reduction sweats. Attempt to assume ahead and guess where diet traps might emerge so you can be prepared with a solid bite or interruption.

Hindrances are made to be survived, so add these outcomes to your weight reduction tool kit and watch those pounds drop off, without rushing.

CHAPTER EIGHT

GENUINE FOOD VERSUS FABRICATED FOOD

It's no coincidence that the fast fire ascend in portliness occurred around a similar time to a great extent reused food varieties came more accessible.

Albeit to a great extent reused food varieties are open, they're loaded with calories, low in supplements and increment your statement of various circumstances.

Then again, genuine food sources are authentically sound and can assist you with getting fitter.

What Are Genuine Food varieties?

Genuine food sources are single-part food sources that are plentiful in nutrients and minerals, warrant synthetic supplements and are significantly stripped down.

There are only numerous Apples, Bananas, Chia seeds, Broccoli, Kale, Berries, Tomatoes, Yams, Earthy coloured rice, Salmon, Entire eggs, and stripped meat. There are loads of genuine food varieties in each nutritional category, so there's a huge range you can integrate into your eating regimen.

Then, at that point, are the motivations behind why genuine food varieties can assist you with shedding pounds.

1. Genuine Food varieties Are Nourishing

The entire, stripped production line and monster food sources are loaded with nutrients and minerals that are perfect for your well-being.

Once more, reused food varieties are low in micronutrients and can expand your statement of medical issues.

Reused food varieties can decelerate weight reduction in more than one way.

For example, an eating routine of reused food varieties that don't give sufficient iron could influence your capacity to work out, since iron is expected to move oxygen around your body. This would restrict your capacity to consume workouts.

An eating regimen low in supplements may likewise help you from getting in shape by causing you to feel less full after eating.

One investigation of 786 individuals looked at entertainers ' interests in completeness when they were on a low-micronutrient diet versus a high-micronutrient diet.

Almost 80 of the entertainers felt more full after reflections on the high-micronutrient diet, without a doubt however they were eating more modest calories than on the low-micronutrient diet.

While you're attempting to expand your contribution of supplements, eating genuine food sources is the best approach. They contain various supplements fragile to track down in a solitary enhancement, including plant composites, nutrients and minerals.

Supplements in entire food varieties likewise will quite often work all the more together and are bound to endure processing than supplements.

Focus point

An eating routine wealthy in supplements might assist with fat misfortune by culminating nutritive shortcomings and decreasing yearning.

2. They're Loaded With Protein

Protein is the main supplement for fat misfortune.

It helps increment your digestion, decrease yearning and influences the result of chemicals that assist with controlling weight.

Your food decisions for protein are similarly essentially as significant as how significant you eat. Genuine food sources are a superior wellspring of protein since they aren't intensely reused.

Food handling can make a few fundamental amino acids harder to process and less accessible to the body. These incorporate lysine, tryptophan, methionine and cysteine.

This is because proteins smoothly answer with sugars and fats associated with handling to frame an intricate mix.

Entire wellsprings of protein are for the most part progressed in protein and lower in calories, which improves them for fat misfortune.

For example,3.5 ounces(100 grams) of pork, a genuine food choice, has 21 grams of protein and 145 calories.

In the meantime, a similar quantity of bacon, a reused food, has 12 grams of protein and 458 calories.

Natural food wellsprings of protein incorporate extra cuts of meat, eggs, vegetables and nuts. You can track down an extraordinary rundown of high-protein food varieties in this piece.

Focus point

Protein is the main supplement for fat misfortune. Genuine food varieties are better wellsprings of protein since they're less reused and by and large have further protein and lower fat.

3. Genuine Food varieties Don't Contain Refined Sugars

The normal sugars set up in products of the soil aren't equivalent to refined sugars.

Leafy foods contain normal sugars, yet additionally give different supplements like fibre, nutrients and water, which are requested as a feature of a reasonable eating routine.

Refined sugars, then again, are as often as possible added to reused food varieties. The two most normal kinds of added sugars are high-fructose slop saccharinity and table sugar.

Food sources progressed in refined sugars are much of the time progressed in calories and give more modest medical advantages. Frozen yoghurt, galettes, eyefuls and luxuries are simply numerous culprits.
Eating further of these food sources is connected with stoutness, so if weight reduction is your thing, restricting them is beautiful.

Refined sugars likewise do essentially nothing to keep you full. Concentrates on demonstrating the way that a high contribution of refined sugar can expand the result of the yearning chemical ghrelin and cover the cerebrum's capacity to encourage you.
Since genuine food sources contain no refined sugars, they're a vastly improved decision for weight reduction.

Focus point
Genuine food sources don't contain added sugar and have different supplements that are perfect for your

well-being. Food sources excellently in added sugar are for the most part progressed in calories, aren't as filling and increment your alarming message of heftiness.

4. They're Progressed In Dissolvable Fiber

Dissolvable fibre gives various medical advantages, and one of them is abetting weight reduction.

It blends in with water in the stomach to frame a thick gel and may decrease your hunger by decelerating the development of food through the stomach.

Another way responsible fibre might diminish craving is by influencing the result of chemicals engaged with overseeing hunger.

Studies have set up that liable fibre might drop the result of chemicals that make you unfilled.

In addition, it might likewise build the result of chemicals that keep you feeling full, including cholecystokinin, glucagon-such as peptide-1 and peptide YY.

Genuine food varieties by and large have further responsible fiber than reused food sources. Incredible wellsprings of liable fibre incorporate sap, flaxseeds, yams and oranges.

Perfectly, intend to eat sufficient fibre every day from entire food sources since they give different supplements. all things considered, individuals who battle to eat sufficient fibre could likewise find an enhancement valuable.

Focus point

Solvent fibre might assist you with shedding pounds by diminishing your hunger. Extraordinary genuine food wellsprings of responsible fibre incorporate yams, sap, and products of the soil.

5. Genuine Food varieties Contain Polyphenols

Plant food sources contain polyphenols, which have cancer prevention agent divides that help cover against grumblings and may likewise assist you with getting thinner.

Polyphenols can be separated into different orders, including lignans, stilbenoids and flavonoids.

One specific flavonoid that is connected with weight reduction is epigallocatechin gallate(EGCG). It's set up in green tea and gives various of its proposed benefits.

For example, EGCG might assist with broadening the merchandise of chemicals engaged with fat consumption, like norepinephrine, by hindering their breakdown.

Various examinations show that drinking green tea might assist you with consuming more calories. Most extreme individuals in these examinations consume 3 - 4 further calories day to day, so the normal individual who consumes 2,000 calories each day could consume 60 - 80 repetitive calories.

Focus point
Genuine food sources are an extraordinary wellspring of polyphenols, which are manufacturing plant bits with cell reinforcement packages. Some polyphenols may assist with fat misfortune, like epigallocatechin gallate in green tea.

6. Genuine Food sources Don't Contain Fake Trans Fats
In any case, it's that counterfeit trans fats are awful for your well-being and your midsection, Assuming there's one thing sustenance researchers settle on.

These fats are naturally made by siphoning hydrogen bits into vegetable materials, transforming them from fluid to strong.

This treatment was intended to expand the timeframe of realistic usability of reused food varieties, similar to eyefuls, galettes and doughnuts(26). Various investigations have set up that continually eating counterfeit trans fats hurts your well-being and your waist.

Overall, contrasted with monkeys that ate an eating regimen wealthy in monounsaturated fats, like those set up in olive oil painting.

Strangely, all the fat the monkeys acquired went directly to their gut region, which expands the danger of heart objections, type 2 diabetes and other medical issues.

Luckily, genuine food sources don't contain counterfeit trans fats.

A few sources like meat, veal and heavenly messenger truly do contain normal trans fats. various investigations have set up that, not at all like counterfeit trans fats, regular trans fats are harmless.

Focus point

Fake trans fats increase fat and lift the danger of various hazardous circumstances. Genuine food varieties don't contain fake trans fats.

7. They'll Assist You With eating further drowsily

Taking the time and eating languidly is a piece of weight reduction exhortation that is habitually disregarded.

In any case, eating drowsily gives your cerebrum a further chance to reuse your food info and feta when it's full.

Genuine food sources can assist with decelerating your eating since they for the most part have a firmer, more wiry surface that should be chewed more. This basic activity can assist you with getting in shape by encouraging you to eat a lower quantity of food.

For one case, an investigation of 30 men set up the people who chewed each nibble multiple times and ate around 12 lower foods than the individuals who chewed multiple times.

The concentrate additionally showed that entertainers who chewed each chomp multiple times had lower craving chemical ghrelin in their blood after the wreck and further of the completeness chemicals glucagon-suchlike peptide-1 and cholecystokinin.

Focus point
Genuine food varieties can assist you with eating drowsily by making you nibble more. This might diminish your hunger and leave you happy with lower food.

8. Genuine Food Sources Might Decrease Sugar Jones

The greatest test with weight reduction oftentimes isn't the eating regimen, yet rather resisting ones for tacky food varieties.
This is difficult, particularly if you're somebody who eats a ton of desserts.

Natural products like berries and tombstones natural products can give a better sweet fix, fulfilling pleasantness when you begin diminishing your sugar input.

It's likewise perfect to know your taste inclinations don't endure ever and can change as you change your eating regimen. Eating further genuine food varieties might help your taste kids adjust and your sugar jones might drop over the long run, or possibly disappear.

Focus point
Genuine food sources give a better sweet fix. Eating further genuine food sources might help your taste kids adjust, diminishing Jones after some time.

9. You Can Eat More Food and nevertheless Get fitter
One major benefit of genuine food sources is that they by and large fill further off a plate than reused food sources while outfitting more modest calories.

This is because various genuine food varieties contain a decent piece of air and water, which is without calories.

For example, 226 grams(a portion of a pound) of cooked pumpkin contains around 45 calories and would take up a lesser part of your plate than a solitary cut of throws containing 66 calories.

Food varieties with more modest calories and further volume can top you off more than food varieties with additional calories and lower volume. They stretch the stomach, and the stomach's stretch receptors motion the mind to quit eating.

The cerebrum likewise answers by creating chemicals that diminish your craving and increment your enthusiasm for completeness.
Extraordinary food decisions that are high in volume yet low in calories incorporate pumpkin, cucumbers, berries and air-popped popcorn.

Focus point
Genuine food varieties for the most part have more modest calories per gram than reused food varieties. Extraordinary food varieties that are high in volume incorporate pumpkin, cucumbers, berries and air-popped popcorn.

10. They'll Diminish Your Utilization to a Great extent Reused Food sources

Heftiness is a colossal medical condition around the world, with over 1.9 billion individuals beyond 18 years old named either fat or fat.

Strangely, the quick-fire ascend in breadth occurred around the very time that generally reused food varieties came widely accessible.

An outline of these progressions should be visible in one review that noticed the patterns to a great extent reused food utilization and stoutness in Sweden somewhere in the range of 1960 and 2010.

The review set up a 142 expansion in the utilization of generally reused food, a 315 expansion in soft drink utilization and a 367 expansion in the utilization of to a great extent reused snacks, comparable to chips and delights.

Simultaneously, stoutness rates further than multiplied, from 5 in 1980 to north of 11 in 2010.

Eating further genuine food diminishes the contribution of to a great extent reused food sources that give numerous supplements, are loaded with void calories and increment the danger of various wellbeing related conditions.

Focus point

Eating all the more genuine food varieties decreases the contribution of reused food varieties, diminishing your alarming message of portliness.

11. Genuine Food varieties Will Assist You With making a Way of life Change

Following an accident diet might assist you with getting fit snappily, yet keeping it off is the greatest test.

Most extreme accidents slim down to assist you with arriving at your thing by limiting nutrition types or radically decreasing calories.

Tragically, on the off chance that their way of eating is aware you can't keep up with the long haul, likewise keeping weight out can be a battle.

That is where eating an eating routine wealthy in genuine food varieties can assist you with getting thinner and keeping up with those advantages long haul. It moves your concentration to pursue food decisions that are better for your waist and your well-being.

Albeit this way of eating could mean weight reduction takes more time to do, you're bound to keep up with what you lose because you've made a life-altering event.

Focus point
Moving your concentration to eat further genuine food sources, as opposed to following an eating regimen, may assist you with getting thinner and keeping it off long haul.

CONCLUSION

An eating routine wealthy in genuine food varieties is perfect for your well-being and can likewise assist you with getting fitter.

Genuine food sources are more healthful, contain more modest calories and are more filling than most extremely reused food sources.

By essentially supplanting reused food varieties in your eating regimen with additional genuine food sources, you can make a major stride towards carrying on with a better life.

Likewise, fostering a propensity for eating genuine food varieties — instead of following a transient eating routine — will make it simpler for you to keep up with long-haul fat misfortune.

The sleek method for getting in shape is to make unending life-altering events to be better. Be that as it may, you ought to look for help from medical care professionals who can assist with directing you toward the most secure and best weight reduction styles, Assuming you're dubious about an eating regimen.

What would it be a good idea for me to consider? Ensure that your eating routine is as yet solid and adjusted. In this way, focus on eating a great many vegetables, organic products, spare proteins, sound fats, and entire grains.

You ought to eat to the point of giving you the energy you want to do your diurnal assignments, including exercise. Certain individuals track down that IF designs like substitute day fasting can make them battle to focus, so the 168 examples could be simpler to make due.

In general, you ought to eat a solid eating routine by decreasing your contribution of added sugars, impregnated fat, and to a great extent reused food varieties. Be that as it may, if you truly do decide to attempt IF likewise ensure it's reasonable for yourself and focus on a fair eating routine when you do eat.

www.ingramcontent.com/pod-product-compliance
Lightning Source LLC
Chambersburg PA
CBHW060953260726
48661CB00005B/1863